Body Shaping for Women
Fitness Journal

by
William Murrell

Bloomington, IN 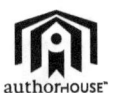 Milton Keynes, UK

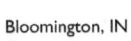

AuthorHouse™
1663 Liberty Drive, Suite 200
Bloomington, IN 47403
www.authorhouse.com
Phone: 1-800-839-8640

AuthorHouse™ UK Ltd.
500 Avebury Boulevard
Central Milton Keynes, MK9 2BE
www.authorhouse.co.uk
Phone: 08001974150

First published by AuthorHouse 5/16/2006

ISBN: 1-4259-2389-5 (sc)

Printed in the United States of America
Bloomington, Indiana

This book is printed on acid-free paper.

Strongly Advised.

This program is not a cure or an aide to counter act any medical recommendations. Before using this program it is strongly suggested that you seek or visit a physician if you have any medical problems or handicaps.

Table of Contents

Introduction

One question a lot of people would like to know is how you introduce yourself to a new change. Is it basic will power, determination, desire, or just mind over matter? The answer is, all the above and this booklet is designed to encourage those among anything else to initiate the power of determination and to show you how to develop. It is to take you from your current basic or intermediate understanding to an elevated enterprise of working out. This guided documentation is to help introduce you to the concept and designed patterns associated with the human anatomy and to allow you to chronicalize your achievements over a period of time, giving you a broader perspective than you would get from a day-to-day memory. The book can be used as a yardstick by which to measure your performance in the gym or life thus pointing out the paths of strengths and weaknesses. Life as we see it now is a fast pace foot race, but rather it should be a happy and healthy journey to well being. A healthy body is everything now. If need be, take a look over your left shoulder at the competition of fit models, movie stars, gym hunks, swimsuit models and give yourself that extra push towards excellence. The examples of those who met untimely ends because the body didn't matter remind us that the finish line can be anywhere. There is no deadline quite like death, so you may as well go ahead and become a healthy and fit person while you still can. Take care of your body. You are the only one who can.

The Facts about Muscles

The human body as we know is distinctive and magnificently designed with more than 600 separate muscles. Each muscle does only two things:
1. **Contract** when being used and
2. **Expand** when resting.

The **skeletal muscle** is the continuous muscle that we can see and feel when in motion. When body builders work out to increase muscle mass the skeletal muscle is what is being used. The skeletal muscle is the muscle attach to the skeleton and come in pairs to move the bone in one direction and the other to move it back to its origin. These muscles usually contract voluntarily.

Uniquely enough the skeletal muscles are all made of the same biological materials. It's a type of muscle fiber that is elastic and somewhat like a rubber band when in motion. There are hundreds of fibers that make up each muscle. In conjunction of muscle fibers we show to have three different types of muscles within the body:
1. **Smooth**
2. **Cardiac** and
3. **Skeletal**

These are muscles of which body builders mainly train. Smooth muscles are muscles we have no control over of which the brain tells these muscles what to do and cardiac muscle of course is the heart muscle which works involuntarily.

The skeletal muscles as we described earlier also come in a variety of sizes and shapes to allow us to do many types of jobs and activities. They give our body the strength it needs to lift, hold and push things. We also have to take in consideration that all body types are not the same and have different shapes as well as different maneuvering capabilities which bring me to another careful consideration of working out.

These three body types are call

1) **<u>Endomorph</u>** - the larger and fleshier body type that tend to be on the overweight side like fat or pair shape
2) **<u>Mesomorph</u>** - the robust muscular body-build type like an athlete with broad shoulders, narrow waists, and broad hips
3) **<u>Ectomorph</u>** - the skinny or lean body type with distinct bone structure, the model type.

These three body types can vary even if someone else look similar you.

The human body is a miraculous anatomical machine with the incredible ability to renew and replenish itself at any time when drained by using its own built in biomechanical system.

In one specialized area we can see for decades how the body has been transformed out of its natural anatomical structure to a more boisterous physique. Free weight for instance, has enabled us to strive beyond our own natural body weight in many ways by aggressively exploring, amending and challenging the working muscles individually or consecutively. In either case the body has shown beneficial result from the intense training. So remember, all forms of exercise will involve some type of weightlifting or reconditioning aerobics.

There is also a difference between what we call aerobic and anaerobic training. The aerobic training include activities such as jogging, bike riding, stair master, etc., and anaerobic include isometric activities such as weightlifting. They are both essentially weightlifting in a sense when it comes to bodybuilding.

The only anaerobic exercise most weightlifters focus on is chest, back, shoulders, arms, abs, thighs and calves.

The important aspect to build muscles is to be consistent in your performance. If you use the **on** again, **off** again technique to exercising it will only prove to be more disappointing than anything else. To get results, you need to commit yourself **faithfully to** exercising!

Also remember muscles are trained to think as well as we do. You need to constantly change your routine to keep them confused. Never repeat the same exercise over and over in the same order, switch things around each time. Also never strain your muscle when they are fatigue but train them in the manner that will give you a return of gratification.

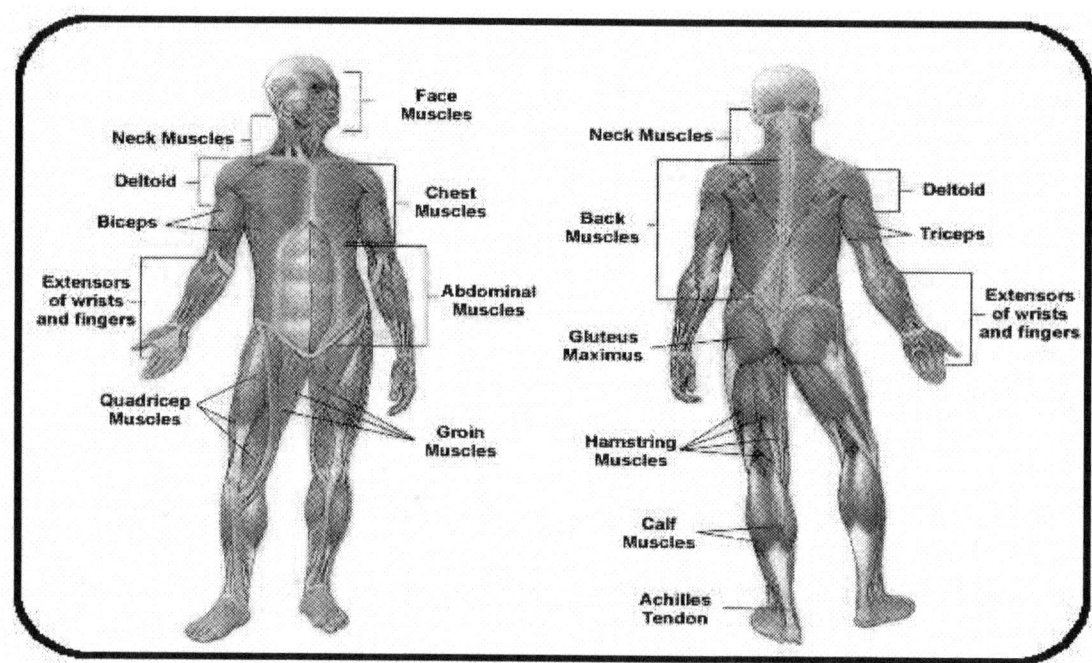

This information as expressed earlier is merely a tool to get you started, and help you adjust your personal program to fit your goals and body chemistry. As you become more knowledgeable about the gyms equipment (what it does), the amount of weight to use, the number of repetitions per set, and rest period between work outs, you will be able to create a training regimen that works best for you.

Proper Eating Is the Key to Being Fit

The proper dietary consumption is needed in order for our body to reach its potential goal. We eat for the necessary reason to live but we also eat to consume the natural resources for growth. The body is a systematic temple that takes distinctive shapes whether we want it to or not, so if it's going to fluctuate why not participate with the outcome of it by exercising.

As study shows the Dept of Health and some nutritionist say that a healthy balanced diet is based on the six basic food groups but in body shaping a careful selection and the amount of diet is the key to maintaining a healthy look:

- Sugars and fats

- Dairy Products

- Meat, fish, poultry, dry beans, eggs, nuts

- Fruit

- Vegetables

- Bread, cereal, rice, pasta

Why do we gain or lose weight?

Well in a study of calories if you eat more than your body burns, on an average you will put on about 1 pound of body weight. If your body burns up more than you eat, you will lose about 1 pound in weight.

The only factor that influences how we gain, lose or maintain weight is the number of calories we consume in compared with the number of calories our body uses. This is also true for the athlete as it is for everyone else.

Here is an illustration to give you an idea of the consumption of calories.

Calories consumed	Calories burned	
3,500 calories	3,000 calories	Gain weight
3,500 calories	4,000 calories	Lose weight
3,500 calories	3,500 calories	Stable weight

The Change of Eating Habits

Eating excessively is another one of our profound weaknesses of being out of shape. At any moment we can begin to eat just for the sake of doing it without consciously thinking about it, for example when reading or watching TV. To begin a serious workout program you have to be willing and determine to make a sacrifice for a limited time to reach your desirable goal.

The guidelines expressed in the booklet isn't just for athletes and the robust, but also for those who desire to control their weight a little better by trying to maintain a level of protein or increase in protein to keep from losing as well as lower the intake of carbohydrates. For training you don't have to eat large meals, but it is recommended that you eat something within 45 minutes after training. A lot of people get positive results with a high-protein shake but too much at one time will become a waste to the body and be disposed of in natural human exportations, also be aware of extremely high sugar and carbohydrates intake in juice drinks because it could be stored as fat and demean the reason for working out. Take body measurements and weight before working out and then slowly experiment with the proportions of food, carbohydrates, protein and fat to find out what works best for you. Here are some things to try and avoid during the process of your workout.......

1. **Saturated fat-** like butter, whole-fat cheese, whole milk and other high calorie dairy products.

2. **Tran fats-** like margarine, cakes, pies, frostings and fried foods (especially if you are trying to loose weight and lean up).

3. **High-sodium foods** –like spices, pretzels, vinegar chips and etc., which causes the body to retain a lot of water and could also help in the long run to lower your risk of high blood pressure, heart attack or stroke thus causing the body to be much healthier.

4. **Fat-free cakes, pies, brownies and cookies** – because most of these items are extremely high in sugar, and as mention earlier could turn to fat composites. One or two cakes as a treat for sticking to the program isn't bad just don't make it a routine habit.

More Helpful Hints to Eating Well

- By eating slow usually means eating less and staying in control without feeling deprived or over eating.

- If you're planning to dine at a restaurant for the evening, eat sensibly throughout the day because it is much easier to stay in control.

- When you finish eating move away from the table because if you tend to linger even though you're no longer hungry, leftovers can tempt you to keep nibbling and overstuff yourself.

- When possible during the day eat a small snack before going to a party to help you avoid eating more than you should once you're there. Remember you're working out to look good.

- If you are not sure about the food being served at a party or social event you can bring your own healthy snack as a second option.

Good health means eating right and exercising. Poor nutrition is just the opposite that's why we must learn the importants of our consuming resources. We must keep in mind the amount we eat, the type of foods we eat, when to eat and how to eat like every two to three hours to keep the metabolism active.

The Program for Working Out to Lose or Tone

This program is typically designed for the purpose of gaining weight, toning up or losing weight all according to the way you want to look. It is also just a tool of some ideas about working out.

Lose or Tone:

__Losing Weight__ - Start with a smaller to medium amount of weight and perform a burn out routine such as 20 reps, then 15 reps, then 10 reps, then 10 reps, and continue this workout for your complete body exercise upper and lower. Also at the end of each workout do cardio, the bike, treadmill or stair master for at least 20 to 30 minutes.

__Toning__ - Start with a medium amount of weight and do 10 reps for four sets. You can increase the weight or keep it the same as long as you do the 10 reps for each set. Last, do abs - obliques (side to side), crunches or leg raises, 50 to 100 everyday.

- Be true to yourself, practice proper range of motion, be consistent and <u>don't cheat.</u>

- Be smart with your workout; don't try to be superman or inhuman starting out with a lot of weights because you don't want to look embarrassed.

- Don't let anyone push you beyond your ability or limits, work at your goal gradually. Your body won't change overnight.

- If you can't increase in weights each week, go back to the previous week and do the same routine but don't stay at the same weights throughout the course of the program.

- **EXERCISE AT YOUR OWN RISK.**

Training Program   (5 Days a week)

Monday	Tuesday	Wednesday	Thursday	Friday

Monday

- Chest
- Biceps
- Triceps

Tuesday

- Cardio

Wednesday

- Quads
- Hamstrings
- Calves

Thursday

- Cardio

Friday

- Back
- Shoulders
- Traps

Monday, Tuesday, Wednesday, Thursday, Friday

- Abdominals
- Cardio

Aerobic Exercises of choice

Stationary Bike, Treadmill, Aerobic classes, Racquetball, Jump rope, Ski machine, Jogging, Jumping jacks, Boxing, Basketball, Walking, Stair stepper, Swimming, Volleyball, Water polo, Rock climbing, Football, and etc.

Chest Exercises

1. **<u>Bench Press</u>**: Lie flat on the bench with your feet flat on the floor. Hold the bar with your hands slightly wider than the width of your shoulders. Lift the weight to the position directly above your chest with arms straight but not locked. Slowly lower the weight until it touches the area just above your nipples. Then slowly lift the bar up until your arms are straight but not locked. Repeat the process until your sets are complete.

2. **<u>Incline Bench Press</u>**: Lie back on the incline bench with it set at 30 degrees. Grasp the weight with your hands slightly wider than the width of your shoulders. Lower the weight bar to your upper chest. Then return the weight to its starting position and repeat the process until your sets are complete.

3. **<u>Incline Fly</u>**: Lie back on an incline bench with it set at 30 degrees and hold the dumbbells with your palms facing each other. Keep your elbows bent slightly so that your forearms are at a 45-degree angle. Lower your arms slowly moving the weight outward at a 90-degree angle above your torso. Move the weights out in an arc fashion. Stop when you reached the bottom then follow the same path back up, bringing the weights together at the top. While doing this exercise don't start with weights that are too heavy.

4. **<u>Decline Bench Press</u>**: Lie back on the decline bench and grasp the weight bar with your hands slightly wider than the width of your shoulders. Lower the weight bar to the bottom base of your chest below the nipple area and lift the bar back up to the starting position slowly to complete the set then repeat until your sets are complete.

5. **<u>Dips</u>**: Grip the parallel dipping bars holding yourself up in a vertical position. Bend your legs with your feet up behind you, and then lower yourself with elbows bent slightly backward and outward during your descent. When you've gone as deep as you can go, slowly raise yourself back to the upright starting position. Don't lower yourself too fast because that will defeat the purpose.

Back Exercises

1. **Wide-grip Pull-down:** Sit down at the pull-down hammer machine and grasp the bar with your hands placed wider than the width of your shoulders, preferably near the end of the bar but not at the very end. Pull the bar down to touch your chest and slowly return the bar back to the starting position. Repeat this process until sets are complete.

2. **Bent-over Barbell Row:** Stand holding a weight bar with a wide grip, palms facing forward and your arms extended downward in front of you. Bend your knees slightly and lean forward placing yourself at a 45-degree angle. Keep your back arched, with your head up and chest out. Lift the weight bar up to your upper abdomen and slowly return it back to the starting position, then repeat this process until you are finished.

3. **Dumbbell Rows:** Lean forward with your body at a 45 degree angle bracing yourself on something or use a bench placing your left knee and left hand on it while your right foot is flat on the floor, keeping your body at a 45 degree angle. Grasp a dumbbell of your choice and pull upward as far as you can go. Keep your back parallel with the floor at all times careful not the twist your torso during the sets. Continue this routine for both sides of the back.

4. **Seated Cable Rows:** Sit on the bench with both legs slightly arched in front of you. Grasp the weight bar, V-bar, B- bar, or U-bar and pull it towards your abdomen in a clean smooth fashion. Don't lean backward with the weight like you're in the process of lying down. Keep your torso up in a 45 degree fashion and bring the weight to you and slowly return it back to the starting position. Continue this until your sets are done.

Leg Exercises

1. <u>Leg Press</u>: Sit and lean back on the pad of the leg press machine. Place your feet shoulder-width apart on the foot platform. Push on the platform equally with both feet and straighten your legs pushing the weight away from you but don't lock them. Then return the platform back to the starting position.

2. <u>Barbell Squat</u>: Stand with your feet about shoulder-width apart and bar across your upper back or what we call traps, holding the bar with both hands. Slowly bend your knees in a decent until your thighs are parallel with the floor then in the same fashion return to the starting position. If you can't reach this point you may be using too much weight. Decrease the weight and try it again. Be sure to keep your head straight ahead throughout the process.

3. <u>Lunges</u>: Pick up a set of dumbbells of your choice with palms facing inward and stand with both feet about 12 inches apart. One at a time take the right foot and step forward until the right thigh is parallel with the floor then push yourself back to the starting position and repeat the process with opposite side. Keep the torso straight and not bent forward.

4. <u>Leg Extensions</u>: Sit and lean back on the pad of the leg machine. Place your legs behind the pad at a 40 to 45 degree angle and select the desirable amount to weight. Once you are comfortable in this position extend your legs forward until they are almost straight but not lock then return them to the starting position and repeat the process until your set is done.

5. <u>Hamstrings</u>: Seated machine. Sit and lean back on the pad of the leg machine. Select the desirable amount to weight and place your legs straight out in front of you with your legs on top of the pads. Lock your legs in with the brace bar then pull pad down with lower legs then back in the starting position and continue this until your sets are complete.

6. <u>Calf Raises</u>: Seated machine. Sit on the machine at a 45 degree angle and place your knees under the pad and lift with lower limbs and then back down and continue until desired sets are complete.

7. <u>Donkey Calf Raises</u>: This routine can be done at home. Lean the body forward at a 45 degree angle bracing yourself on something, have someone to sit on your lower back area like riding a horse and lift lower legs up and down until desired sets are complete.

Biceps Exercises

1. <u>Standing Barbell Curl</u>: Stand straight with both your palms facing forward. Grasp the barbell with the weight hanging down in front of you. Slowly lift the bar to your shoulder level and then return to the weight to the starting position and repeat until you are finished your sets.

2. <u>Seated Preacher Curl</u>: Sit at a preacher bench and grab the weight bar with our palms up. Put your tricep area on the pad and don't allow them to move out of balance during the routine. Extend your arm forward and then curl the weight back up toward your shoulders in a slow and steady motion. Continue this until you have finished your sets.

3. <u>Dumbbell Alternating Curl</u>: Stand straight in an upright position holding a pair of dumbbells at your side with palms facing inward to your thighs. Slowly in a steady fashion lift the weight up (one arm at a time), toward your shoulders and then bring it back to it's starting position. Try to keep your body steady with no swaying while lifting. It's important to your bicep workout.

4. <u>Alternating Cable Curl</u>: Stand straight facing the cable machine, keeping your upper body in an upright position. Grasp the D-ring for cable with your palm facing forward. Slowly in a steady fashion lift the weight up (one arm at a time), toward your shoulders and then bring it back to its starting position. Try to keep your body steady with no swaying while lifting at all times.

Triceps Exercises

1. **<u>Seated Dumbbell Triceps Extension</u>:** Sit on a bench with the seat at a 90-degree angle. Hold the dumbbell behind your head so it is level with the floor. Interlock your fingers while holding the dumbbell then slowly raise the dumbbell above your head and slowly lower the weight back down behind your head as far as you can go. Repeat this process until your routine is completed.

2. **<u>Triceps Kickback</u>:** Lean forward with your body at a 90-degree angle. Take the cable or dumbbell of your choice in one hand and raise your arm in a 90-degree angle so that your tricep is parallel to the floor. In a slow control fashion move the dumbbell backward until it is almost fully extended. Lower the weight back to the starting position with the arm at a 90-degree angle and start all over again until done then switch arms.

3. **<u>Cable Extension</u>:** Grasp the cable D-ring standing upright facing the machine with palm facing forward. Slowly, pull the cable down to fully extend the arm while concentrating on the triceps then slowly raise your arm back up at a 90-degree angle. Continue this until finish and then switch arms. Maintain good posture while performing this routine.

Shoulder Exercises

1. <u>Military Press</u>: Sit on the bench at a 90-degree angle with dumbbells of your choice. Lift the dumbbells in each hand over your shoulders with your palms facing forward. Slowly lift both arms straight up above your shoulders and then return back to starting position. Continue this until your set is done.

2. <u>Front Cable Raises</u>: Stand in front of a cable machine completely upright with the D-ring or cable to your side. Grasp the D-ring with your palm facing backward and down by your side. Keeping your arm straight with a slight bend, raise the cable straight out in front of you until your arm is parallel with the floor. When your set is complete switch arms.

3. <u>Front Dumbbell Raises</u>: Stand with a pair of dumbbells hanging in front of you with your palms facing your thighs. Place feet shoulder width apart and then with one arm at a time raise the dumbbells until your arms are level or parallel with the floor. Continue this until your set is complete.

4. <u>Side Dumbbell Raises</u>: Stand with a pair of dumbbells of your choice hanging at your side with your palms facing inward to your thighs. Place feet shoulder width apart and then with both arms straight, raise the weight outward from your side until they are parallel to the floor and then lower them back down to the starting position. Do this until you have finished your set.

Sample Ideas of Workout Routines

Mass & Tone do <u>4 Sets</u>   /   Lose/Tone do <u>3 Sets</u>

Mass (Heavy Weight) **Increase weight each set**	**Tone (Med Weight)** **Add 10 lbs per set or stay**	**Lose/Tone (Med Weight)** **Drop 5 lbs per rep**
1. 15 (Set 1) 15 (Set 2) 15 (Set 3) 15 (Set 4)	1. 10 (Set 1) 10 (Set 2) 10 (Set 3) 10 (Set 4)	1. 15, 12, 10, 10 (Set 1) 15, 12, 10, 10 (Set 2) 12, 12, 10, 10 (Set 3)
2. 15 (Set 1) 15 (Set 2) 15 (Set 3) 12 (Set 4)	2. 12 (Set 1) 12 (Set 2) 12 (Set 3) 12 (Set 4)	2. 15, 15, 15, 15 (Set 1) 15, 12, 10, 10 (Set 2) 12, 12, 12, 12 (Set 3)
3. 15 (Set 1) 12 (Set 2) 12 (Set 3) 12 (Set 4)	3. 12 (Set 1) 12 (Set 2) 10 (Set 3) 10 (Set 4)	3. 12, 12, 12, 12 (Set 1) 12, 10, 10, 10 (Set 2) 10, 10, 10, 10 (Set 3)
4. 12 (Set 1) 12 (Set 2) 12 (Set 3) 12 (Set 4)	4. 15 (Set 1) 12 (Set 2) 12 (Set 3) 12 (Set 4)	4. 12, 10, 10, 10 (Set 1) 10, 10, 8, 8 (Set 2) 10, 8, 6, 6 (Set 3)
5. 15 (Set 1) 12 (Set 2) 10 (Set 3) 10 (Set 4)	5. 15 (Set 1) 15 (Set 2) 10 (Set 3) 10 (Set 4)	5. 10, 10, 8, 8 (Set 1) 10, 10, 8, 8 (Set 2) 10, 8, 8, 6 (Set 3)
6. 12 (Set 1) 12 (Set 2) 10 (Set 3) 10 (Set 4)		

Diagram of Fitness Chart

Number of Sets(4) - Example 15,15,15,12

The exercise Example # 1 Bench Press

The amount of weight

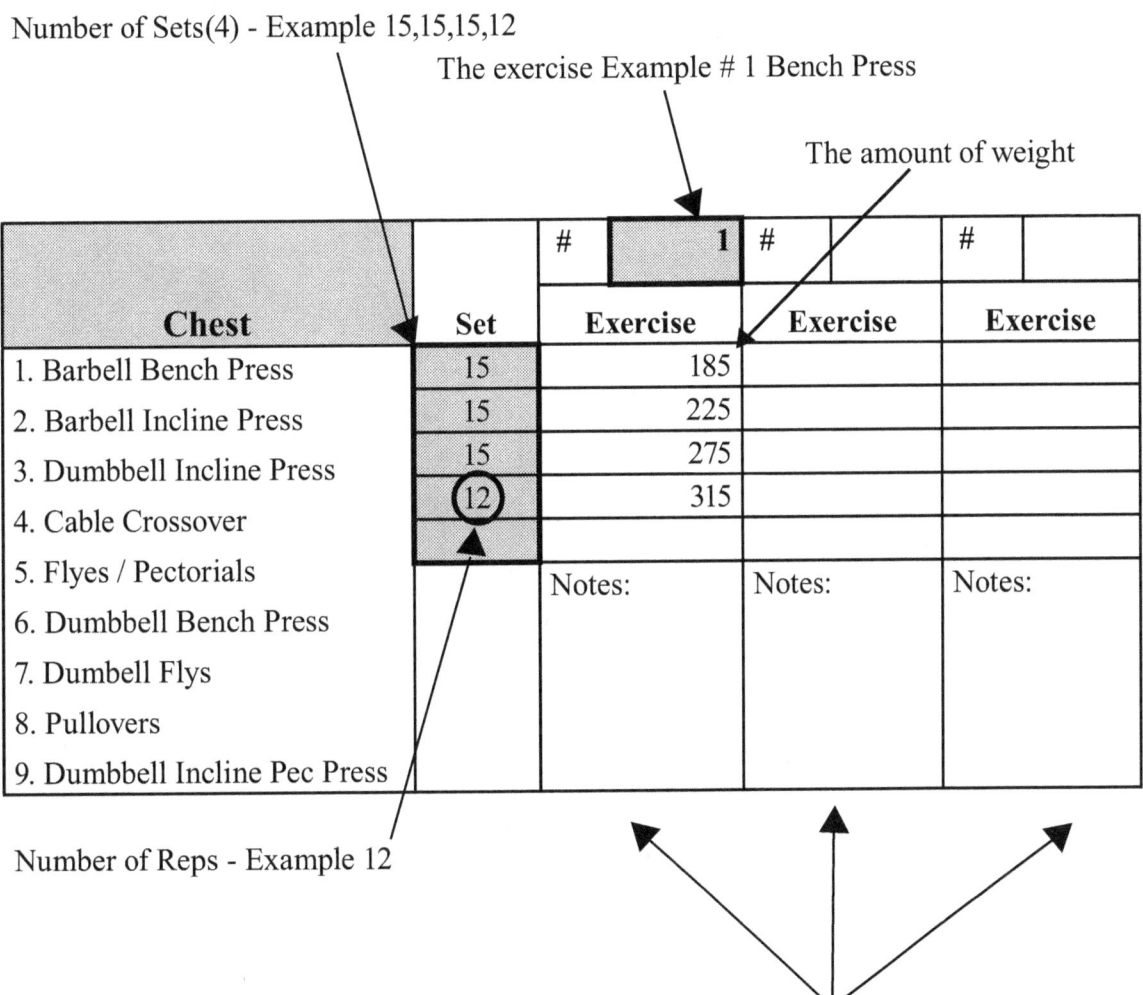

Chest	Set	#	1	#		#	
		Exercise		Exercise		Exercise	
1. Barbell Bench Press	15	185					
2. Barbell Incline Press	15	225					
3. Dumbbell Incline Press	15	275					
4. Cable Crossover	12	315					
5. Flyes / Pectorials							
6. Dumbbell Bench Press		Notes:		Notes:		Notes:	
7. Dumbell Flys							
8. Pullovers							
9. Dumbbell Incline Pec Press							

Number of Reps - Example 12

Three boxes for three different exercise for the muscle group

Daily Fitness Assessment

Week _____ Date _____ / _____ / _____

Upper Body Workout

Chest	Set	# Exercise		# Exercise		# Exercise	
1. Barbell Bench Press							
2. Barbell Incline Press							
3. Dumbbell Incline Press							
4. Cable Crossover							
5. Flyes / Pectorials							
6. Dumbbell Bench Press							
7. Dumbell Flys or Pullovers		Notes:		Notes:		Notes:	

Biceps	Set	# Exercise		# Exercise		# Exercise	
1. Alternating Cable Curls							
2. Seated Concentration Curls							
3. Hammer Curls							
4. Standing EZ Curls							
5. Dumbbell Curls							
6. Barbell Curls		Notes:		Notes:		Notes:	

Triceps	Set	# Exercise		# Exercise		# Exercise	
1. Seated Tricep Presses							
2. Triceps Kickbacks							
3. Triceps Pushdowns							
4. Bench Dips							
5. Alternating Standing Extensions							
6. Reverse Tricep Presses							
7. Overhead Bumbell Extensions		Notes:		Notes:		Notes:	

Abdominals	Set	# Exercise		# Exercise		# Exercise	
1. Flat Bench Leg Raises							
2. Bent Knee Raises							
3. Machine Crunches							
4. Lying Twisting Crunches							
5. Seated Twisting Crunches							
6. Single Plate Twisting Crunches		Notes:		Notes:		Notes:	

Daily Fitness Assessment

Week _____   Date _____/_____/_____

Upper Body Workout

Chest	Set	# Exercise		# Exercise		# Exercise	
1. Barbell Bench Press							
2. Barbell Incline Press							
3. Dumbbell Incline Press							
4. Cable Crossover							
5. Flyes / Pectorials							
6. Dumbbell Bench Press							
7. Dumbell Flys or Pullovers		Notes:		Notes:		Notes:	

Biceps	Set	# Exercise		# Exercise		# Exercise	
1. Alternating Cable Curls							
2. Seated Concentration Curls							
3. Hammer Curls							
4. Standing EZ Curls							
5. Dumbbell Curls							
6. Barbell Curls		Notes:		Notes:		Notes:	

Triceps	Set	# Exercise		# Exercise		# Exercise	
1. Seated Tricep Presses							
2. Triceps Kickbacks							
3. Triceps Pushdowns							
4. Bench Dips							
5. Alternating Standing Extensions							
6. Reverse Tricep Presses							
7. Overhead Bumbell Extensions		Notes:		Notes:		Notes:	

Abdominals	Set	# Exercise		# Exercise		# Exercise	
1. Flat Bench Leg Raises							
2. Bent Knee Raises							
3. Machine Crunches							
4. Lying Twisting Crunches							
5. Seated Twisting Crunches							
6. Single Plate Twisting Crunches		Notes:		Notes:		Notes:	

Daily Fitness Assessment

Week _____   Date _____/_____/_____

Upper Body Workout

Chest	Set	#	Exercise	#	Exercise	#	Exercise
1. Barbell Bench Press							
2. Barbell Incline Press							
3. Dumbbell Incline Press							
4. Cable Crossover							
5. Flyes / Pectorials							
6. Dumbbell Bench Press							
7. Dumbell Flys or Pullovers			Notes:		Notes:		Notes:

Biceps	Set	#	Exercise	#	Exercise	#	Exercise
1. Alternating Cable Curls							
2. Seated Concentration Curls							
3. Hammer Curls							
4. Standing EZ Curls							
5. Dumbbell Curls							
6. Barbell Curls			Notes:		Notes:		Notes:

Triceps	Set	#	Exercise	#	Exercise	#	Exercise
1. Seated Tricep Presses							
2. Triceps Kickbacks							
3. Triceps Pushdowns							
4. Bench Dips							
5. Alternating Standing Extensions							
6. Reverse Tricep Presses							
7. Overhead Bumbell Extensions			Notes:		Notes:		Notes:

Abdominals	Set	#	Exercise	#	Exercise	#	Exercise
1. Flat Bench Leg Raises							
2. Bent Knee Raises							
3. Machine Crunches							
4. Lying Twisting Crunches							
5. Seated Twisting Crunches							
6. Single Plate Twisting Crunches			Notes:		Notes:		Notes:

Daily Fitness Assessment

Week _____   Date _____/_____/_____

Upper Body Workout

Chest	Set	# Exercise		# Exercise		# Exercise	
1. Barbell Bench Press							
2. Barbell Incline Press							
3. Dumbbell Incline Press							
4. Cable Crossover							
5. Flyes / Pectorials							
6. Dumbbell Bench Press							
7. Dumbell Flys or Pullovers		Notes:		Notes:		Notes:	

Biceps	Set	# Exercise		# Exercise		# Exercise	
1. Alternating Cable Curls							
2. Seated Concentration Curls							
3. Hammer Curls							
4. Standing EZ Curls							
5. Dumbbell Curls							
6. Barbell Curls		Notes:		Notes:		Notes:	

Triceps	Set	# Exercise		# Exercise		# Exercise	
1. Seated Tricep Presses							
2. Triceps Kickbacks							
3. Triceps Pushdowns							
4. Bench Dips							
5. Alternating Standing Extensions							
6. Reverse Tricep Presses							
7. Overhead Bumbell Extensions		Notes:		Notes:		Notes:	

Abdominals	Set	# Exercise		# Exercise		# Exercise	
1. Flat Bench Leg Raises							
2. Bent Knee Raises							
3. Machine Crunches							
4. Lying Twisting Crunches							
5. Seated Twisting Crunches							
6. Single Plate Twisting Crunches		Notes:		Notes:		Notes:	

Daily Fitness Assessment

Week _____   Date _____/_____/_____

Upper Body Workout

Chest	Set	# Exercise		# Exercise		# Exercise	
1. Barbell Bench Press							
2. Barbell Incline Press							
3. Dumbbell Incline Press							
4. Cable Crossover							
5. Flyes / Pectorials							
6. Dumbbell Bench Press							
7. Dumbell Flys or Pullovers		Notes:		Notes:		Notes:	

Biceps	Set	# Exercise		# Exercise		# Exercise	
1. Alternating Cable Curls							
2. Seated Concentration Curls							
3. Hammer Curls							
4. Standing EZ Curls							
5. Dumbbell Curls							
6. Barbell Curls		Notes:		Notes:		Notes:	

Triceps	Set	# Exercise		# Exercise		# Exercise	
1. Seated Tricep Presses							
2. Triceps Kickbacks							
3. Triceps Pushdowns							
4. Bench Dips							
5. Alternating Standing Extensions							
6. Reverse Tricep Presses							
7. Overhead Bumbell Extensions		Notes:		Notes:		Notes:	

Abdominals	Set	# Exercise		# Exercise		# Exercise	
1. Flat Bench Leg Raises							
2. Bent Knee Raises							
3. Machine Crunches							
4. Lying Twisting Crunches							
5. Seated Twisting Crunches							
6. Single Plate Twisting Crunches		Notes:		Notes:		Notes:	

Daily Fitness Assessment

Week _____   **Date** _____/_____/_____

Upper Body Workout

Chest	Set	# Exercise		# Exercise		# Exercise	
1. Barbell Bench Press							
2. Barbell Incline Press							
3. Dumbbell Incline Press							
4. Cable Crossover							
5. Flyes / Pectorials							
6. Dumbbell Bench Press							
7. Dumbell Flys or Pullovers		Notes:		Notes:		Notes:	

Biceps	Set	# Exercise		# Exercise		# Exercise	
1. Alternating Cable Curls							
2. Seated Concentration Curls							
3. Hammer Curls							
4. Standing EZ Curls							
5. Dumbbell Curls							
6. Barbell Curls		Notes:		Notes:		Notes:	

Triceps	Set	# Exercise		# Exercise		# Exercise	
1. Seated Tricep Presses							
2. Triceps Kickbacks							
3. Triceps Pushdowns							
4. Bench Dips							
5. Alternating Standing Extensions							
6. Reverse Tricep Presses							
7. Overhead Bumbell Extensions		Notes:		Notes:		Notes:	

Abdominals	Set	# Exercise		# Exercise		# Exercise	
1. Flat Bench Leg Raises							
2. Bent Knee Raises							
3. Machine Crunches							
4. Lying Twisting Crunches							
5. Seated Twisting Crunches							
6. Single Plate Twisting Crunches		Notes:		Notes:		Notes:	

Daily Fitness Assessment

Week _____   Date _____/_____/_____

Upper Body Workout

Chest	Set	#	Exercise	#	Exercise	#	Exercise
1. Barbell Bench Press							
2. Barbell Incline Press							
3. Dumbbell Incline Press							
4. Cable Crossover							
5. Flyes / Pectorials							
6. Dumbbell Bench Press							
7. Dumbell Flys or Pullovers			Notes:		Notes:		Notes:

Biceps	Set	#	Exercise	#	Exercise	#	Exercise
1. Alternating Cable Curls							
2. Seated Concentration Curls							
3. Hammer Curls							
4. Standing EZ Curls							
5. Dumbbell Curls							
6. Barbell Curls			Notes:		Notes:		Notes:

Triceps	Set	#	Exercise	#	Exercise	#	Exercise
1. Seated Tricep Presses							
2. Triceps Kickbacks							
3. Triceps Pushdowns							
4. Bench Dips							
5. Alternating Standing Extensions							
6. Reverse Tricep Presses							
7. Overhead Bumbell Extensions			Notes:		Notes:		Notes:

Abdominals	Set	#	Exercise	#	Exercise	#	Exercise
1. Flat Bench Leg Raises							
2. Bent Knee Raises							
3. Machine Crunches							
4. Lying Twisting Crunches							
5. Seated Twisting Crunches							
6. Single Plate Twisting Crunches			Notes:		Notes:		Notes:

Daily Fitness Assessment

Week _____   Date _____/_____/_____

Upper Body Workout

Chest	Set	# Exercise		# Exercise		# Exercise	
1. Barbell Bench Press							
2. Barbell Incline Press							
3. Dumbbell Incline Press							
4. Cable Crossover							
5. Flyes / Pectorials							
6. Dumbbell Bench Press							
7. Dumbell Flys or Pullovers		Notes:		Notes:		Notes:	

Biceps	Set	# Exercise		# Exercise		# Exercise	
1. Alternating Cable Curls							
2. Seated Concentration Curls							
3. Hammer Curls							
4. Standing EZ Curls							
5. Dumbbell Curls							
6. Barbell Curls		Notes:		Notes:		Notes:	

Triceps	Set	# Exercise		# Exercise		# Exercise	
1. Seated Tricep Presses							
2. Triceps Kickbacks							
3. Triceps Pushdowns							
4. Bench Dips							
5. Alternating Standing Extensions							
6. Reverse Tricep Presses							
7. Overhead Bumbell Extensions		Notes:		Notes:		Notes:	

Abdominals	Set	# Exercise		# Exercise		# Exercise	
1. Flat Bench Leg Raises							
2. Bent Knee Raises							
3. Machine Crunches							
4. Lying Twisting Crunches							
5. Seated Twisting Crunches							
6. Single Plate Twisting Crunches		Notes:		Notes:		Notes:	

Daily Fitness Assessment

Week _____   Date _____/_____/_____

Upper Body Workout

Chest	Set	#	Exercise	#	Exercise	#	Exercise
1. Barbell Bench Press							
2. Barbell Incline Press							
3. Dumbbell Incline Press							
4. Cable Crossover							
5. Flyes / Pectorials							
6. Dumbbell Bench Press							
7. Dumbell Flys or Pullovers			Notes:		Notes:		Notes:

Biceps	Set	#	Exercise	#	Exercise	#	Exercise
1. Alternating Cable Curls							
2. Seated Concentration Curls							
3. Hammer Curls							
4. Standing EZ Curls							
5. Dumbbell Curls							
6. Barbell Curls			Notes:		Notes:		Notes:

Triceps	Set	#	Exercise	#	Exercise	#	Exercise
1. Seated Tricep Presses							
2. Triceps Kickbacks							
3. Triceps Pushdowns							
4. Bench Dips							
5. Alternating Standing Extensions							
6. Reverse Tricep Presses							
7. Overhead Bumbell Extensions			Notes:		Notes:		Notes:

Abdominals	Set	#	Exercise	#	Exercise	#	Exercise
1. Flat Bench Leg Raises							
2. Bent Knee Raises							
3. Machine Crunches							
4. Lying Twisting Crunches							
5. Seated Twisting Crunches							
6. Single Plate Twisting Crunches			Notes:		Notes:		Notes:

Daily Fitness Assessment

Week _____   Date _____/_____/_____

Upper Body Workout

Chest	Set	# Exercise		# Exercise		# Exercise	
1. Barbell Bench Press							
2. Barbell Incline Press							
3. Dumbbell Incline Press							
4. Cable Crossover							
5. Flyes / Pectorials							
6. Dumbbell Bench Press							
7. Dumbell Flys or Pullovers		Notes:		Notes:		Notes:	

Biceps	Set	# Exercise		# Exercise		# Exercise	
1. Alternating Cable Curls							
2. Seated Concentration Curls							
3. Hammer Curls							
4. Standing EZ Curls							
5. Dumbbell Curls							
6. Barbell Curls		Notes:		Notes:		Notes:	

Triceps	Set	# Exercise		# Exercise		# Exercise	
1. Seated Tricep Presses							
2. Triceps Kickbacks							
3. Triceps Pushdowns							
4. Bench Dips							
5. Alternating Standing Extensions							
6. Reverse Tricep Presses							
7. Overhead Bumbell Extensions		Notes:		Notes:		Notes:	

Abdominals	Set	# Exercise		# Exercise		# Exercise	
1. Flat Bench Leg Raises							
2. Bent Knee Raises							
3. Machine Crunches							
4. Lying Twisting Crunches							
5. Seated Twisting Crunches							
6. Single Plate Twisting Crunches		Notes:		Notes:		Notes:	

Daily Fitness Assessment

Week _____   Date _____ / _____ / _____

Upper Body Workout

Chest	Set	#	Exercise	#	Exercise	#	Exercise
1. Barbell Bench Press							
2. Barbell Incline Press							
3. Dumbbell Incline Press							
4. Cable Crossover							
5. Flyes / Pectorials							
6. Dumbbell Bench Press							
7. Dumbell Flys or Pullovers			Notes:		Notes:		Notes:

Biceps	Set	#	Exercise	#	Exercise	#	Exercise
1. Alternating Cable Curls							
2. Seated Concentration Curls							
3. Hammer Curls							
4. Standing EZ Curls							
5. Dumbbell Curls							
6. Barbell Curls			Notes:		Notes:		Notes:

Triceps	Set	#	Exercise	#	Exercise	#	Exercise
1. Seated Tricep Presses							
2. Triceps Kickbacks							
3. Triceps Pushdowns							
4. Bench Dips							
5. Alternating Standing Extensions							
6. Reverse Tricep Presses							
7. Overhead Bumbell Extensions			Notes:		Notes:		Notes:

Abdominals	Set	#	Exercise	#	Exercise	#	Exercise
1. Flat Bench Leg Raises							
2. Bent Knee Raises							
3. Machine Crunches							
4. Lying Twisting Crunches							
5. Seated Twisting Crunches							
6. Single Plate Twisting Crunches			Notes:		Notes:		Notes:

Daily Fitness Assessment

Week _____   **Date** _____/_____/_____

Upper Body Workout

Chest	Set	# Exercise		# Exercise		# Exercise	
1. Barbell Bench Press							
2. Barbell Incline Press							
3. Dumbbell Incline Press							
4. Cable Crossover							
5. Flyes / Pectorials							
6. Dumbbell Bench Press							
7. Dumbell Flys or Pullovers		Notes:		Notes:		Notes:	

Biceps	Set	# Exercise		# Exercise		# Exercise	
1. Alternating Cable Curls							
2. Seated Concentration Curls							
3. Hammer Curls							
4. Standing EZ Curls							
5. Dumbbell Curls							
6. Barbell Curls		Notes:		Notes:		Notes:	

Triceps	Set	# Exercise		# Exercise		# Exercise	
1. Seated Tricep Presses							
2. Triceps Kickbacks							
3. Triceps Pushdowns							
4. Bench Dips							
5. Alternating Standing Extensions							
6. Reverse Tricep Presses							
7. Overhead Bumbell Extensions		Notes:		Notes:		Notes:	

Abdominals	Set	# Exercise		# Exercise		# Exercise	
1. Flat Bench Leg Raises							
2. Bent Knee Raises							
3. Machine Crunches							
4. Lying Twisting Crunches							
5. Seated Twisting Crunches							
6. Single Plate Twisting Crunches		Notes:		Notes:		Notes:	

Daily Fitness Assessment

Week _____   **Date** _____/_____/_____

Upper Body Workout

Chest	Set	# Exercise		# Exercise		# Exercise	
1. Barbell Bench Press							
2. Barbell Incline Press							
3. Dumbbell Incline Press							
4. Cable Crossover							
5. Flyes / Pectorials							
6. Dumbbell Bench Press							
7. Dumbell Flys or Pullovers		Notes:		Notes:		Notes:	

Biceps	Set	# Exercise		# Exercise		# Exercise	
1. Alternating Cable Curls							
2. Seated Concentration Curls							
3. Hammer Curls							
4. Standing EZ Curls							
5. Dumbbell Curls							
6. Barbell Curls		Notes:		Notes:		Notes:	

Triceps	Set	# Exercise		# Exercise		# Exercise	
1. Seated Tricep Presses							
2. Triceps Kickbacks							
3. Triceps Pushdowns							
4. Bench Dips							
5. Alternating Standing Extensions							
6. Reverse Tricep Presses							
7. Overhead Bumbell Extensions		Notes:		Notes:		Notes:	

Abdominals	Set	# Exercise		# Exercise		# Exercise	
1. Flat Bench Leg Raises							
2. Bent Knee Raises							
3. Machine Crunches							
4. Lying Twisting Crunches							
5. Seated Twisting Crunches							
6. Single Plate Twisting Crunches		Notes:		Notes:		Notes:	

Daily Fitness Assessment

Week _____   Date _____/_____/_____

Upper Body Workout

Chest	Set	# Exercise		# Exercise		# Exercise	
1. Barbell Bench Press							
2. Barbell Incline Press							
3. Dumbbell Incline Press							
4. Cable Crossover							
5. Flyes / Pectorials							
6. Dumbbell Bench Press							
7. Dumbell Flys or Pullovers		Notes:		Notes:		Notes:	

Biceps	Set	# Exercise		# Exercise		# Exercise	
1. Alternating Cable Curls							
2. Seated Concentration Curls							
3. Hammer Curls							
4. Standing EZ Curls							
5. Dumbbell Curls							
6. Barbell Curls		Notes:		Notes:		Notes:	

Triceps	Set	# Exercise		# Exercise		# Exercise	
1. Seated Tricep Presses							
2. Triceps Kickbacks							
3. Triceps Pushdowns							
4. Bench Dips							
5. Alternating Standing Extensions							
6. Reverse Tricep Presses							
7. Overhead Bumbell Extensions		Notes:		Notes:		Notes:	

Abdominals	Set	# Exercise		# Exercise		# Exercise	
1. Flat Bench Leg Raises							
2. Bent Knee Raises							
3. Machine Crunches							
4. Lying Twisting Crunches							
5. Seated Twisting Crunches							
6. Single Plate Twisting Crunches		Notes:		Notes:		Notes:	

43

Daily Fitness Assessment

Week _____   **Date** _____/_____/_____

Upper Body Workout

Chest	Set	# Exercise		# Exercise		# Exercise	
1. Barbell Bench Press							
2. Barbell Incline Press							
3. Dumbbell Incline Press							
4. Cable Crossover							
5. Flyes / Pectorials							
6. Dumbbell Bench Press							
7. Dumbell Flys or Pullovers		Notes:		Notes:		Notes:	

Biceps	Set	# Exercise		# Exercise		# Exercise	
1. Alternating Cable Curls							
2. Seated Concentration Curls							
3. Hammer Curls							
4. Standing EZ Curls							
5. Dumbbell Curls							
6. Barbell Curls		Notes:		Notes:		Notes:	

Triceps	Set	# Exercise		# Exercise		# Exercise	
1. Seated Tricep Presses							
2. Triceps Kickbacks							
3. Triceps Pushdowns							
4. Bench Dips							
5. Alternating Standing Extensions							
6. Reverse Tricep Presses							
7. Overhead Bumbell Extensions		Notes:		Notes:		Notes:	

Abdominals	Set	# Exercise		# Exercise		# Exercise	
1. Flat Bench Leg Raises							
2. Bent Knee Raises							
3. Machine Crunches							
4. Lying Twisting Crunches							
5. Seated Twisting Crunches							
6. Single Plate Twisting Crunches		Notes:		Notes:		Notes:	

Daily Fitness Assessment for

Week _____   **Date** _____/_____/_____

Lower Body Workout

Quadriceps	Set	#	Exercise	#	Exercise	#	Exercise
1. Barbell Squats							
2. Leg Presses							
3. Leg Extensions							
4. Hack Squats							
5. Lunges			Notes:		Notes:		Notes:

Hamstrings	Set	#	Exercise	#	Exercise	#	Exercise
1. Dumbbell Lunges							
2. Lying Leg Curls							
3. Staight-Leg Deadlifts							
4. Standing Leg Curls			Notes:		Notes:		Notes:

Calves	Set	#	Exercise	#	Exercise	#	Exercise
1. Seated Calf Raises							
2. Standing Heel Raises							
3. Donkey Calf Raises							
4. One Leg Calf Raises			Notes:		Notes:		Notes:

Abdominals	Set	#	Exercise	#	Exercise	#	Exercise
1. Flat Bench Leg Raises							
2. Bent Knee Raises							
3. Machine Crunches							
4. Lying Twisting Crunches							
5. Seated Twisting Crunches							
6. Single Plate Twisting Crunches			Notes:		Notes:		Notes:

Daily Fitness Assessment for

Week _____   Date _____/_____/_____

Lower Body Workout

Quadriceps	Set	#	Exercise	#	Exercise	#	Exercise
1. Barbell Squats							
2. Leg Presses							
3. Leg Extensions							
4. Hack Squats							
5. Lunges			Notes:		Notes:		Notes:

Hamstrings	Set	#	Exercise	#	Exercise	#	Exercise
1. Dumbbell Lunges							
2. Lying Leg Curls							
3. Staight-Leg Deadlifts							
4. Standing Leg Curls			Notes:		Notes:		Notes:

Calves	Set	#	Exercise	#	Exercise	#	Exercise
1. Seated Calf Raises							
2. Standing Heel Raises							
3. Donkey Calf Raises							
4. One Leg Calf Raises			Notes:		Notes:		Notes:

Abdominals	Set	#	Exercise	#	Exercise	#	Exercise
1. Flat Bench Leg Raises							
2. Bent Knee Raises							
3. Machine Crunches							
4. Lying Twisting Crunches							
5. Seated Twisting Crunches							
6. Single Plate Twisting Crunches			Notes:		Notes:		Notes:

Daily Fitness Assessment for

Week _____   Date _____/_____/_____

Lower Body Workout

Quadriceps	Set	# Exercise	# Exercise	# Exercise
1. Barbell Squats				
2. Leg Presses				
3. Leg Extensions				
4. Hack Squats				
5. Lunges		Notes:	Notes:	Notes:

Hamstrings	Set	# Exercise	# Exercise	# Exercise
1. Dumbbell Lunges				
2. Lying Leg Curls				
3. Staight-Leg Deadlifts				
4. Standing Leg Curls		Notes:	Notes:	Notes:

Calves	Set	# Exercise	# Exercise	# Exercise
1. Seated Calf Raises				
2. Standing Heel Raises				
3. Donkey Calf Raises				
4. One Leg Calf Raises		Notes:	Notes:	Notes:

Abdominals	Set	# Exercise	# Exercise	# Exercise
1. Flat Bench Leg Raises				
2. Bent Knee Raises				
3. Machine Crunches				
4. Lying Twisting Crunches				
5. Seated Twisting Crunches				
6. Single Plate Twisting Crunches		Notes:	Notes:	Notes:

Daily Fitness Assessment for

Week _____   **Date** _____/_____/_____

Lower Body Workout

Quadriceps	Set	# Exercise		# Exercise		# Exercise	
1. Barbell Squats							
2. Leg Presses							
3. Leg Extensions							
4. Hack Squats							
5. Lunges		Notes:		Notes:		Notes:	

Hamstrings	Set	# Exercise		# Exercise		# Exercise	
1. Dumbbell Lunges							
2. Lying Leg Curls							
3. Staight-Leg Deadlifts							
4. Standing Leg Curls		Notes:		Notes:		Notes:	

Calves	Set	# Exercise		# Exercise		# Exercise	
1. Seated Calf Raises							
2. Standing Heel Raises							
3. Donkey Calf Raises							
4. One Leg Calf Raises		Notes:		Notes:		Notes:	

Abdominals	Set	# Exercise		# Exercise		# Exercise	
1. Flat Bench Leg Raises							
2. Bent Knee Raises							
3. Machine Crunches							
4. Lying Twisting Crunches							
5. Seated Twisting Crunches							
6. Single Plate Twisting Crunches		Notes:		Notes:		Notes:	

Daily Fitness Assessment for

Week _____ **Date** _____/_____/_____

Lower Body Workout

Quadriceps	Set	# Exercise		# Exercise		# Exercise	
1. Barbell Squats							
2. Leg Presses							
3. Leg Extensions							
4. Hack Squats							
5. Lunges		Notes:		Notes:		Notes:	

Hamstrings	Set	# Exercise		# Exercise		# Exercise	
1. Dumbbell Lunges							
2. Lying Leg Curls							
3. Staight-Leg Deadlifts							
4. Standing Leg Curls		Notes:		Notes:		Notes:	

Calves	Set	# Exercise		# Exercise		# Exercise	
1. Seated Calf Raises							
2. Standing Heel Raises							
3. Donkey Calf Raises							
4. One Leg Calf Raises		Notes:		Notes:		Notes:	

Abdominals	Set	# Exercise		# Exercise		# Exercise	
1. Flat Bench Leg Raises							
2. Bent Knee Raises							
3. Machine Crunches							
4. Lying Twisting Crunches							
5. Seated Twisting Crunches							
6. Single Plate Twisting Crunches		Notes:		Notes:		Notes:	

Daily Fitness Assessment for

Week _____   **Date** _____/_____/_____

Lower Body Workout

Quadriceps	Set	# Exercise	# Exercise	# Exercise
1. Barbell Squats				
2. Leg Presses				
3. Leg Extensions				
4. Hack Squats				
5. Lunges		Notes:	Notes:	Notes:

Hamstrings	Set	# Exercise	# Exercise	# Exercise
1. Dumbbell Lunges				
2. Lying Leg Curls				
3. Staight-Leg Deadlifts				
4. Standing Leg Curls		Notes:	Notes:	Notes:

Calves	Set	# Exercise	# Exercise	# Exercise
1. Seated Calf Raises				
2. Standing Heel Raises				
3. Donkey Calf Raises				
4. One Leg Calf Raises		Notes:	Notes:	Notes:

Abdominals	Set	# Exercise	# Exercise	# Exercise
1. Flat Bench Leg Raises				
2. Bent Knee Raises				
3. Machine Crunches				
4. Lying Twisting Crunches				
5. Seated Twisting Crunches				
6. Single Plate Twisting Crunches		Notes:	Notes:	Notes:

Daily Fitness Assessment for

Week _____   Date _____/_____/_____

Lower Body Workout

Quadriceps	Set	# Exercise	# Exercise	# Exercise
1. Barbell Squats				
2. Leg Presses				
3. Leg Extensions				
4. Hack Squats				
5. Lunges		Notes:	Notes:	Notes:

Hamstrings	Set	# Exercise	# Exercise	# Exercise
1. Dumbbell Lunges				
2. Lying Leg Curls				
3. Staight-Leg Deadlifts				
4. Standing Leg Curls		Notes:	Notes:	Notes:

Calves	Set	# Exercise	# Exercise	# Exercise
1. Seated Calf Raises				
2. Standing Heel Raises				
3. Donkey Calf Raises				
4. One Leg Calf Raises		Notes:	Notes:	Notes:

Abdominals	Set	# Exercise	# Exercise	# Exercise
1. Flat Bench Leg Raises				
2. Bent Knee Raises				
3. Machine Crunches				
4. Lying Twisting Crunches				
5. Seated Twisting Crunches				
6. Single Plate Twisting Crunches		Notes:	Notes:	Notes:

Daily Fitness Assessment for

Week _____   **Date** _____/_____/_____

Lower Body Workout

Quadriceps	Set	#	Exercise	#	Exercise	#	Exercise
1. Barbell Squats							
2. Leg Presses							
3. Leg Extensions							
4. Hack Squats							
5. Lunges			Notes:		Notes:		Notes:

Hamstrings	Set	#	Exercise	#	Exercise	#	Exercise
1. Dumbbell Lunges							
2. Lying Leg Curls							
3. Staight-Leg Deadlifts							
4. Standing Leg Curls			Notes:		Notes:		Notes:

Calves	Set	#	Exercise	#	Exercise	#	Exercise
1. Seated Calf Raises							
2. Standing Heel Raises							
3. Donkey Calf Raises							
4. One Leg Calf Raises			Notes:		Notes:		Notes:

Abdominals	Set	#	Exercise	#	Exercise	#	Exercise
1. Flat Bench Leg Raises							
2. Bent Knee Raises							
3. Machine Crunches							
4. Lying Twisting Crunches							
5. Seated Twisting Crunches							
6. Single Plate Twisting Crunches			Notes:		Notes:		Notes:

Daily Fitness Assessment for

Week _____   **Date** _____/_____/_____

Lower Body Workout

Quadriceps	Set	#		#		#	
		Exercise		**Exercise**		**Exercise**	
1. Barbell Squats							
2. Leg Presses							
3. Leg Extensions							
4. Hack Squats							
5. Lunges		Notes:		Notes:		Notes:	

Hamstrings	Set	#		#		#	
		Exercise		**Exercise**		**Exercise**	
1. Dumbbell Lunges							
2. Lying Leg Curls							
3. Staight-Leg Deadlifts							
4. Standing Leg Curls		Notes:		Notes:		Notes:	

Calves	Set	#		#		#	
		Exercise		**Exercise**		**Exercise**	
1. Seated Calf Raises							
2. Standing Heel Raises							
3. Donkey Calf Raises							
4. One Leg Calf Raises		Notes:		Notes:		Notes:	

Abdominals	Set	#		#		#	
		Exercise		**Exercise**		**Exercise**	
1. Flat Bench Leg Raises							
2. Bent Knee Raises							
3. Machine Crunches							
4. Lying Twisting Crunches							
5. Seated Twisting Crunches							
6. Single Plate Twisting Crunches		Notes:		Notes:		Notes:	

Daily Fitness Assessment for

Week _____   Date _____/_____/_____

Lower Body Workout

Quadriceps	Set	# Exercise	# Exercise	# Exercise
1. Barbell Squats				
2. Leg Presses				
3. Leg Extensions				
4. Hack Squats				
5. Lunges		Notes:	Notes:	Notes:

Hamstrings	Set	# Exercise	# Exercise	# Exercise
1. Dumbbell Lunges				
2. Lying Leg Curls				
3. Staight-Leg Deadlifts				
4. Standing Leg Curls		Notes:	Notes:	Notes:

Calves	Set	# Exercise	# Exercise	# Exercise
1. Seated Calf Raises				
2. Standing Heel Raises				
3. Donkey Calf Raises				
4. One Leg Calf Raises		Notes:	Notes:	Notes:

Abdominals	Set	# Exercise	# Exercise	# Exercise
1. Flat Bench Leg Raises				
2. Bent Knee Raises				
3. Machine Crunches				
4. Lying Twisting Crunches				
5. Seated Twisting Crunches				
6. Single Plate Twisting Crunches		Notes:	Notes:	Notes:

Daily Fitness Assessment for

Week _____   Date _____/_____/_____

Lower Body Workout

Quadriceps	Set	# Exercise		# Exercise		# Exercise	
1. Barbell Squats							
2. Leg Presses							
3. Leg Extensions							
4. Hack Squats							
5. Lunges		Notes:		Notes:		Notes:	

Hamstrings	Set	# Exercise		# Exercise		# Exercise	
1. Dumbbell Lunges							
2. Lying Leg Curls							
3. Staight-Leg Deadlifts							
4. Standing Leg Curls		Notes:		Notes:		Notes:	

Calves	Set	# Exercise		# Exercise		# Exercise	
1. Seated Calf Raises							
2. Standing Heel Raises							
3. Donkey Calf Raises							
4. One Leg Calf Raises		Notes:		Notes:		Notes:	

Abdominals	Set	# Exercise		# Exercise		# Exercise	
1. Flat Bench Leg Raises							
2. Bent Knee Raises							
3. Machine Crunches							
4. Lying Twisting Crunches							
5. Seated Twisting Crunches							
6. Single Plate Twisting Crunches		Notes:		Notes:		Notes:	

Daily Fitness Assessment for

Week _____   Date _____/_____/_____

Lower Body Workout

Quadriceps	Set	# Exercise	# Exercise	# Exercise
1. Barbell Squats				
2. Leg Presses				
3. Leg Extensions				
4. Hack Squats				
5. Lunges		Notes:	Notes:	Notes:

Hamstrings	Set	# Exercise	# Exercise	# Exercise
1. Dumbbell Lunges				
2. Lying Leg Curls				
3. Staight-Leg Deadlifts				
4. Standing Leg Curls		Notes:	Notes:	Notes:

Calves	Set	# Exercise	# Exercise	# Exercise
1. Seated Calf Raises				
2. Standing Heel Raises				
3. Donkey Calf Raises				
4. One Leg Calf Raises		Notes:	Notes:	Notes:

Abdominals	Set	# Exercise	# Exercise	# Exercise
1. Flat Bench Leg Raises				
2. Bent Knee Raises				
3. Machine Crunches				
4. Lying Twisting Crunches				
5. Seated Twisting Crunches				
6. Single Plate Twisting Crunches		Notes:	Notes:	Notes:

Daily Fitness Assessment for

Week _____ **Date** _____/_____/_____

Lower Body Workout

Quadriceps	Set	# Exercise	# Exercise	# Exercise
1. Barbell Squats				
2. Leg Presses				
3. Leg Extensions				
4. Hack Squats				
5. Lunges		Notes:	Notes:	Notes:

Hamstrings	Set	# Exercise	# Exercise	# Exercise
1. Dumbbell Lunges				
2. Lying Leg Curls				
3. Staight-Leg Deadlifts				
4. Standing Leg Curls		Notes:	Notes:	Notes:

Calves	Set	# Exercise	# Exercise	# Exercise
1. Seated Calf Raises				
2. Standing Heel Raises				
3. Donkey Calf Raises				
4. One Leg Calf Raises		Notes:	Notes:	Notes:

Abdominals	Set	# Exercise	# Exercise	# Exercise
1. Flat Bench Leg Raises				
2. Bent Knee Raises				
3. Machine Crunches				
4. Lying Twisting Crunches				
5. Seated Twisting Crunches				
6. Single Plate Twisting Crunches		Notes:	Notes:	Notes:

Daily Fitness Assessment for

Week _____   **Date** _____/_____/_____

Lower Body Workout

Quadriceps	Set	#	Exercise	#	Exercise	#	Exercise
1. Barbell Squats							
2. Leg Presses							
3. Leg Extensions							
4. Hack Squats							
5. Lunges			Notes:		Notes:		Notes:

Hamstrings	Set	#	Exercise	#	Exercise	#	Exercise
1. Dumbbell Lunges							
2. Lying Leg Curls							
3. Staight-Leg Deadlifts							
4. Standing Leg Curls			Notes:		Notes:		Notes:

Calves	Set	#	Exercise	#	Exercise	#	Exercise
1. Seated Calf Raises							
2. Standing Heel Raises							
3. Donkey Calf Raises							
4. One Leg Calf Raises			Notes:		Notes:		Notes:

Abdominals	Set	#	Exercise	#	Exercise	#	Exercise
1. Flat Bench Leg Raises							
2. Bent Knee Raises							
3. Machine Crunches							
4. Lying Twisting Crunches							
5. Seated Twisting Crunches							
6. Single Plate Twisting Crunches			Notes:		Notes:		Notes:

Daily Fitness Assessment for

Week _____ **Date** _____/_____/_____

Lower Body Workout

Quadriceps	Set	# Exercise		# Exercise		# Exercise	
1. Barbell Squats							
2. Leg Presses							
3. Leg Extensions							
4. Hack Squats							
5. Lunges		Notes:		Notes:		Notes:	

Hamstrings	Set	# Exercise		# Exercise		# Exercise	
1. Dumbbell Lunges							
2. Lying Leg Curls							
3. Staight-Leg Deadlifts							
4. Standing Leg Curls		Notes:		Notes:		Notes:	

Calves	Set	# Exercise		# Exercise		# Exercise	
1. Seated Calf Raises							
2. Standing Heel Raises							
3. Donkey Calf Raises							
4. One Leg Calf Raises		Notes:		Notes:		Notes:	

Abdominals	Set	# Exercise		# Exercise		# Exercise	
1. Flat Bench Leg Raises							
2. Bent Knee Raises							
3. Machine Crunches							
4. Lying Twisting Crunches							
5. Seated Twisting Crunches							
6. Single Plate Twisting Crunches		Notes:		Notes:		Notes:	

Daily Fitness Assessment

Week _____   **Date** _____/_____/_____

Upper Body Workout

Back	Set	#	Exercise	#	Exercise	#	Exercise
1. Seated Cable Row							
2. Wide Grip Lat Pulldowns							
3. Front V-Bar Pulldowns							
4. Low Row Extensions							
5. Bar Standing Pulldowns							
6. T- Bar Rows			Notes:		Notes:		Notes:
7. Front Plate Raises							

Shoulders	Set	#	Exercise	#	Exercise	#	Exercise
1. Seated Military Presses							
2. Front Cable Raises							
3. Side Dumbell Lateral Raises							
4. Reverse Flyes							
5. Dumbbell Front Raises							
6. Barbell Upright Rows			Notes:		Notes:		Notes:
7. Side Cable Lateral Raises							

Trapsezius	Set	#	Exercise	#	Exercise	#	Exercise
1. Standing Front Barbell Rows							
2. Standing Rear Barbell Rows							
(Optional for Females)			Notes:		Notes:		Notes:

Abdominals	Set	#	Exercise	#	Exercise	#	Exercise
1. Flat Bench Leg Raises							
2. Bent Knee Raises							
3. Machine Crunches							
4. Lying Twisting Crunches							
5. Seated Twisting Crunches							
6. Single Plate Twisting Crunches							
			Notes:		Notes:		Notes:

Daily Fitness Assessment

Week _____   Date _____ / _____ / _____

Upper Body Workout

Back	Set	# Exercise		# Exercise		# Exercise	
1. Seated Cable Row							
2. Wide Grip Lat Pulldowns							
3. Front V-Bar Pulldowns							
4. Low Row Extensions							
5. Bar Standing Pulldowns							
6. T- Bar Rows							
7. Front Plate Raises		Notes:		Notes:		Notes:	

Shoulders	Set	# Exercise		# Exercise		# Exercise	
1. Seated Military Presses							
2. Front Cable Raises							
3. Side Dumbell Lateral Raises							
4. Reverse Flyes							
5. Dumbbell Front Raises							
6. Barbell Upright Rows							
7. Side Cable Lateral Raises		Notes:		Notes:		Notes:	

Trapsezius	Set	# Exercise		# Exercise		# Exercise	
1. Standing Front Barbell Rows							
2. Standing Rear Barbell Rows							
(Optional for Females)		Notes:		Notes:		Notes:	

Abdominals	Set	# Exercise		# Exercise		# Exercise	
1. Flat Bench Leg Raises							
2. Bent Knee Raises							
3. Machine Crunches							
4. Lying Twisting Crunches							
5. Seated Twisting Crunches							
6. Single Plate Twisting Crunches							
		Notes:		Notes:		Notes:	

Daily Fitness Assessment

Week _____   **Date** _____/_____/_____

Upper Body Workout

Back	Set	# Exercise	# Exercise	# Exercise
1. Seated Cable Row				
2. Wide Grip Lat Pulldowns				
3. Front V-Bar Pulldowns				
4. Low Row Extensions				
5. Bar Standing Pulldowns				
6. T- Bar Rows		Notes:	Notes:	Notes:
7. Front Plate Raises				

Shoulders	Set	# Exercise	# Exercise	# Exercise
1. Seated Military Presses				
2. Front Cable Raises				
3. Side Dumbell Lateral Raises				
4. Reverse Flyes				
5. Dumbbell Front Raises				
6. Barbell Upright Rows		Notes:	Notes:	Notes:
7. Side Cable Lateral Raises				

Trapsezius	Set	# Exercise	# Exercise	# Exercise
1. Standing Front Barbell Rows				
2. Standing Rear Barbell Rows				
(Optional for Females)		Notes:	Notes:	Notes:

Abdominals	Set	# Exercise	# Exercise	# Exercise
1. Flat Bench Leg Raises				
2. Bent Knee Raises				
3. Machine Crunches				
4. Lying Twisting Crunches				
5. Seated Twisting Crunches				
6. Single Plate Twisting Crunches				
		Notes:	Notes:	Notes:

Daily Fitness Assessment

Week _____   **Date** _____/_____/_____

Upper Body Workout

Back	Set	# Exercise		# Exercise		# Exercise	
1. Seated Cable Row							
2. Wide Grip Lat Pulldowns							
3. Front V-Bar Pulldowns							
4. Low Row Extensions							
5. Bar Standing Pulldowns							
6. T- Bar Rows		Notes:		Notes:		Notes:	
7. Front Plate Raises							

Shoulders	Set	# Exercise		# Exercise		# Exercise	
1. Seated Military Presses							
2. Front Cable Raises							
3. Side Dumbell Lateral Raises							
4. Reverse Flyes							
5. Dumbbell Front Raises							
6. Barbell Upright Rows		Notes:		Notes:		Notes:	
7. Side Cable Lateral Raises							

Trapsezius	Set	# Exercise		# Exercise		# Exercise	
1. Standing Front Barbell Rows							
2. Standing Rear Barbell Rows							
(Optional for Females)		Notes:		Notes:		Notes:	

Abdominals	Set	# Exercise		# Exercise		# Exercise	
1. Flat Bench Leg Raises							
2. Bent Knee Raises							
3. Machine Crunches							
4. Lying Twisting Crunches							
5. Seated Twisting Crunches							
6. Single Plate Twisting Crunches		Notes:		Notes:		Notes:	

Daily Fitness Assessment

Week _____   **Date** _____/_____/_____

Upper Body Workout

Back	Set	# Exercise		# Exercise		# Exercise	
1. Seated Cable Row							
2. Wide Grip Lat Pulldowns							
3. Front V-Bar Pulldowns							
4. Low Row Extensions							
5. Bar Standing Pulldowns							
6. T- Bar Rows		Notes:		Notes:		Notes:	
7. Front Plate Raises							

Shoulders	Set	# Exercise		# Exercise		# Exercise	
1. Seated Military Presses							
2. Front Cable Raises							
3. Side Dumbell Lateral Raises							
4. Reverse Flyes							
5. Dumbbell Front Raises							
6. Barbell Upright Rows		Notes:		Notes:		Notes:	
7. Side Cable Lateral Raises							

Trapsezius	Set	# Exercise		# Exercise		# Exercise	
1. Standing Front Barbell Rows							
2. Standing Rear Barbell Rows							
(Optional for Females)		Notes:		Notes:		Notes:	

Abdominals	Set	# Exercise		# Exercise		# Exercise	
1. Flat Bench Leg Raises							
2. Bent Knee Raises							
3. Machine Crunches							
4. Lying Twisting Crunches							
5. Seated Twisting Crunches							
6. Single Plate Twisting Crunches							
		Notes:		Notes:		Notes:	

Daily Fitness Assessment

Week _____   **Date** _____/_____/_____

Upper Body Workout

Back	Set	# Exercise		# Exercise		# Exercise	
1. Seated Cable Row							
2. Wide Grip Lat Pulldowns							
3. Front V-Bar Pulldowns							
4. Low Row Extensions							
5. Bar Standing Pulldowns							
6. T- Bar Rows		Notes:		Notes:		Notes:	
7. Front Plate Raises							

Shoulders	Set	# Exercise		# Exercise		# Exercise	
1. Seated Military Presses							
2. Front Cable Raises							
3. Side Dumbell Lateral Raises							
4. Reverse Flyes							
5. Dumbbell Front Raises							
6. Barbell Upright Rows		Notes:		Notes:		Notes:	
7. Side Cable Lateral Raises							

Trapsezius	Set	# Exercise		# Exercise		# Exercise	
1. Standing Front Barbell Rows							
2. Standing Rear Barbell Rows							
(Optional for Females)		Notes:		Notes:		Notes:	

Abdominals	Set	# Exercise		# Exercise		# Exercise	
1. Flat Bench Leg Raises							
2. Bent Knee Raises							
3. Machine Crunches							
4. Lying Twisting Crunches							
5. Seated Twisting Crunches							
6. Single Plate Twisting Crunches							
		Notes:		Notes:		Notes:	

Daily Fitness Assessment

Week _____   Date _____/_____/_____

Upper Body Workout

Back	Set	# Exercise	# Exercise	# Exercise
1. Seated Cable Row				
2. Wide Grip Lat Pulldowns				
3. Front V-Bar Pulldowns				
4. Low Row Extensions				
5. Bar Standing Pulldowns				
6. T- Bar Rows				
7. Front Plate Raises		Notes:	Notes:	Notes:

Shoulders	Set	# Exercise	# Exercise	# Exercise
1. Seated Military Presses				
2. Front Cable Raises				
3. Side Dumbell Lateral Raises				
4. Reverse Flyes				
5. Dumbbell Front Raises				
6. Barbell Upright Rows				
7. Side Cable Lateral Raises		Notes:	Notes:	Notes:

Trapsezius	Set	# Exercise	# Exercise	# Exercise
1. Standing Front Barbell Rows				
2. Standing Rear Barbell Rows				
(Optional for Females)		Notes:	Notes:	Notes:

Abdominals	Set	# Exercise	# Exercise	# Exercise
1. Flat Bench Leg Raises				
2. Bent Knee Raises				
3. Machine Crunches				
4. Lying Twisting Crunches				
5. Seated Twisting Crunches				
6. Single Plate Twisting Crunches				
		Notes:	Notes:	Notes:

Daily Fitness Assessment

Week _____   **Date** _____/_____/_____

Upper Body Workout

Back	Set	# Exercise		# Exercise		# Exercise	
1. Seated Cable Row							
2. Wide Grip Lat Pulldowns							
3. Front V-Bar Pulldowns							
4. Low Row Extensions							
5. Bar Standing Pulldowns							
6. T- Bar Rows		Notes:		Notes:		Notes:	
7. Front Plate Raises							

Shoulders	Set	# Exercise		# Exercise		# Exercise	
1. Seated Military Presses							
2. Front Cable Raises							
3. Side Dumbell Lateral Raises							
4. Reverse Flyes							
5. Dumbbell Front Raises							
6. Barbell Upright Rows		Notes:		Notes:		Notes:	
7. Side Cable Lateral Raises							

Trapsezius	Set	# Exercise		# Exercise		# Exercise	
1. Standing Front Barbell Rows							
2. Standing Rear Barbell Rows							
(Optional for Females)		Notes:		Notes:		Notes:	

Abdominals	Set	# Exercise		# Exercise		# Exercise	
1. Flat Bench Leg Raises							
2. Bent Knee Raises							
3. Machine Crunches							
4. Lying Twisting Crunches							
5. Seated Twisting Crunches							
6. Single Plate Twisting Crunches							
		Notes:		Notes:		Notes:	

Daily Fitness Assessment

Week _____   Date _____/_____/_____

Upper Body Workout

Back	Set	# Exercise	# Exercise	# Exercise
1. Seated Cable Row				
2. Wide Grip Lat Pulldowns				
3. Front V-Bar Pulldowns				
4. Low Row Extensions				
5. Bar Standing Pulldowns				
6. T- Bar Rows		Notes:	Notes:	Notes:
7. Front Plate Raises				

Shoulders	Set	# Exercise	# Exercise	# Exercise
1. Seated Military Presses				
2. Front Cable Raises				
3. Side Dumbell Lateral Raises				
4. Reverse Flyes				
5. Dumbbell Front Raises				
6. Barbell Upright Rows		Notes:	Notes:	Notes:
7. Side Cable Lateral Raises				

Trapsezius	Set	# Exercise	# Exercise	# Exercise
1. Standing Front Barbell Rows				
2. Standing Rear Barbell Rows				
(Optional for Females)		Notes:	Notes:	Notes:

Abdominals	Set	# Exercise	# Exercise	# Exercise
1. Flat Bench Leg Raises				
2. Bent Knee Raises				
3. Machine Crunches				
4. Lying Twisting Crunches				
5. Seated Twisting Crunches				
6. Single Plate Twisting Crunches		Notes:	Notes:	Notes:

Daily Fitness Assessment

Week _____   **Date** _____/_____/_____

Upper Body Workout

Back	Set	#	Exercise	#	Exercise	#	Exercise
1. Seated Cable Row							
2. Wide Grip Lat Pulldowns							
3. Front V-Bar Pulldowns							
4. Low Row Extensions							
5. Bar Standing Pulldowns							
6. T- Bar Rows			Notes:		Notes:		Notes:
7. Front Plate Raises							

Shoulders	Set	#	Exercise	#	Exercise	#	Exercise
1. Seated Military Presses							
2. Front Cable Raises							
3. Side Dumbell Lateral Raises							
4. Reverse Flyes							
5. Dumbbell Front Raises							
6. Barbell Upright Rows			Notes:		Notes:		Notes:
7. Side Cable Lateral Raises							

Trapsezius	Set	#	Exercise	#	Exercise	#	Exercise
1. Standing Front Barbell Rows							
2. Standing Rear Barbell Rows							
(Optional for Females)			Notes:		Notes:		Notes:

Abdominals	Set	#	Exercise	#	Exercise	#	Exercise
1. Flat Bench Leg Raises							
2. Bent Knee Raises							
3. Machine Crunches							
4. Lying Twisting Crunches							
5. Seated Twisting Crunches							
6. Single Plate Twisting Crunches			Notes:		Notes:		Notes:

Daily Fitness Assessment

Week _____   Date _____ / _____ / _____

Upper Body Workout

Back	Set	# Exercise		# Exercise		# Exercise	
1. Seated Cable Row							
2. Wide Grip Lat Pulldowns							
3. Front V-Bar Pulldowns							
4. Low Row Extensions							
5. Bar Standing Pulldowns							
6. T- Bar Rows		Notes:		Notes:		Notes:	
7. Front Plate Raises							

Shoulders	Set	# Exercise		# Exercise		# Exercise	
1. Seated Military Presses							
2. Front Cable Raises							
3. Side Dumbell Lateral Raises							
4. Reverse Flyes							
5. Dumbbell Front Raises							
6. Barbell Upright Rows		Notes:		Notes:		Notes:	
7. Side Cable Lateral Raises							

Trapsezius	Set	# Exercise		# Exercise		# Exercise	
1. Standing Front Barbell Rows							
2. Standing Rear Barbell Rows							
(Optional for Females)		Notes:		Notes:		Notes:	

Abdominals	Set	# Exercise		# Exercise		# Exercise	
1. Flat Bench Leg Raises							
2. Bent Knee Raises							
3. Machine Crunches							
4. Lying Twisting Crunches							
5. Seated Twisting Crunches							
6. Single Plate Twisting Crunches							
		Notes:		Notes:		Notes:	

Daily Fitness Assessment

Week _____   Date _____/_____/_____

Upper Body Workout

Back	Set	# Exercise		# Exercise		# Exercise	
1. Seated Cable Row							
2. Wide Grip Lat Pulldowns							
3. Front V-Bar Pulldowns							
4. Low Row Extensions							
5. Bar Standing Pulldowns							
6. T- Bar Rows		Notes:		Notes:		Notes:	
7. Front Plate Raises							

Shoulders	Set	# Exercise		# Exercise		# Exercise	
1. Seated Military Presses							
2. Front Cable Raises							
3. Side Dumbell Lateral Raises							
4. Reverse Flyes							
5. Dumbbell Front Raises							
6. Barbell Upright Rows		Notes:		Notes:		Notes:	
7. Side Cable Lateral Raises							

Trapsezius	Set	# Exercise		# Exercise		# Exercise	
1. Standing Front Barbell Rows							
2. Standing Rear Barbell Rows							
(Optional for Females)		Notes:		Notes:		Notes:	

Abdominals	Set	# Exercise		# Exercise		# Exercise	
1. Flat Bench Leg Raises							
2. Bent Knee Raises							
3. Machine Crunches							
4. Lying Twisting Crunches							
5. Seated Twisting Crunches							
6. Single Plate Twisting Crunches		Notes:		Notes:		Notes:	

Daily Fitness Assessment

Week _____   Date _____/_____/_____

Upper Body Workout

Back	Set	#	Exercise	#	Exercise	#	Exercise
1. Seated Cable Row							
2. Wide Grip Lat Pulldowns							
3. Front V-Bar Pulldowns							
4. Low Row Extensions							
5. Bar Standing Pulldowns							
6. T- Bar Rows							
7. Front Plate Raises		Notes:		Notes:		Notes:	

Shoulders	Set	#	Exercise	#	Exercise	#	Exercise
1. Seated Military Presses							
2. Front Cable Raises							
3. Side Dumbell Lateral Raises							
4. Reverse Flyes							
5. Dumbbell Front Raises							
6. Barbell Upright Rows							
7. Side Cable Lateral Raises		Notes:		Notes:		Notes:	

Trapsezius	Set	#	Exercise	#	Exercise	#	Exercise
1. Standing Front Barbell Rows							
2. Standing Rear Barbell Rows							
(Optional for Females)		Notes:		Notes:		Notes:	

Abdominals	Set	#	Exercise	#	Exercise	#	Exercise
1. Flat Bench Leg Raises							
2. Bent Knee Raises							
3. Machine Crunches							
4. Lying Twisting Crunches							
5. Seated Twisting Crunches							
6. Single Plate Twisting Crunches							
		Notes:		Notes:		Notes:	

Daily Fitness Assessment

Week _____   Date _____/_____/_____

Upper Body Workout

Back	Set	# Exercise		# Exercise		# Exercise	
1. Seated Cable Row							
2. Wide Grip Lat Pulldowns							
3. Front V-Bar Pulldowns							
4. Low Row Extensions							
5. Bar Standing Pulldowns							
6. T- Bar Rows							
7. Front Plate Raises		Notes:		Notes:		Notes:	

Shoulders	Set	# Exercise		# Exercise		# Exercise	
1. Seated Military Presses							
2. Front Cable Raises							
3. Side Dumbell Lateral Raises							
4. Reverse Flyes							
5. Dumbbell Front Raises							
6. Barbell Upright Rows							
7. Side Cable Lateral Raises		Notes:		Notes:		Notes:	

Trapsezius	Set	# Exercise		# Exercise		# Exercise	
1. Standing Front Barbell Rows							
2. Standing Rear Barbell Rows							
(Optional for Females)		Notes:		Notes:		Notes:	

Abdominals	Set	# Exercise		# Exercise		# Exercise	
1. Flat Bench Leg Raises							
2. Bent Knee Raises							
3. Machine Crunches							
4. Lying Twisting Crunches							
5. Seated Twisting Crunches							
6. Single Plate Twisting Crunches							
		Notes:		Notes:		Notes:	

Daily Fitness Assessment

Week _____   **Date** _____/_____/_____

Upper Body Workout

Back	Set	# Exercise		# Exercise		# Exercise	
1. Seated Cable Row							
2. Wide Grip Lat Pulldowns							
3. Front V-Bar Pulldowns							
4. Low Row Extensions							
5. Bar Standing Pulldowns							
6. T- Bar Rows		Notes:		Notes:		Notes:	
7. Front Plate Raises							

Shoulders	Set	# Exercise		# Exercise		# Exercise	
1. Seated Military Presses							
2. Front Cable Raises							
3. Side Dumbell Lateral Raises							
4. Reverse Flyes							
5. Dumbbell Front Raises							
6. Barbell Upright Rows		Notes:		Notes:		Notes:	
7. Side Cable Lateral Raises							

Trapsezius	Set	# Exercise		# Exercise		# Exercise	
1. Standing Front Barbell Rows							
2. Standing Rear Barbell Rows							
(Optional for Females)		Notes:		Notes:		Notes:	

Abdominals	Set	# Exercise		# Exercise		# Exercise	
1. Flat Bench Leg Raises							
2. Bent Knee Raises							
3. Machine Crunches							
4. Lying Twisting Crunches							
5. Seated Twisting Crunches							
6. Single Plate Twisting Crunches		Notes:		Notes:		Notes:	

Daily Fitness Assessment

Total Body Workout

	#		#		#	
Cardio		Time		Time		Time
1. Stationary Bike						
2. Treadmill						
3. Aerobic classes						
4. Racquetball						
5. Jump rope						
6. Ski machine						
7. Jogging						
8. Jumping jacks						
9. Boxing						
10. Basketball						
11. Walking						
12. Stair stepper						
13. Swimming						
14. Volleyball						
15. Water polo						
16. Rock climbing	Notes:		Notes:		Notes:	
17. Football						

Daily Fitness Assessment

Total Body Workout

Date _____   Date _____   Date _____

Cardio	#	Time	#	Time	#	Time
1. Stationary Bike						
2. Treadmill						
3. Aerobic classes						
4. Racquetball						
5. Jump rope						
6. Ski machine						
7. Jogging						
8. Jumping jacks						
9. Boxing						
10. Basketball						
11. Walking						
12. Stair stepper						
13. Swimming						
14. Volleyball						
15. Water polo						
16. Rock climbing	Notes:		Notes:		Notes:	
17. Football						

Daily Fitness Assessment

Total Body Workout

	Date _____		Date _____		Date _____	
Cardio	#	Time	#	Time	#	Time
1. Stationary Bike						
2. Treadmill						
3. Aerobic classes						
4. Racquetball						
5. Jump rope						
6. Ski machine						
7. Jogging						
8. Jumping jacks						
9. Boxing						
10. Basketball						
11. Walking						
12. Stair stepper						
13. Swimming						
14. Volleyball						
15. Water polo						
16. Rock climbing	Notes:		Notes:		Notes:	
17. Football						

Daily Fitness Assessment

Total Body Workout

	Date _____		Date _____		Date _____	
	#		#		#	
Cardio		Time		Time		Time
1. Stationary Bike						
2. Treadmill						
3. Aerobic classes						
4. Racquetball						
5. Jump rope						
6. Ski machine						
7. Jogging						
8. Jumping jacks						
9. Boxing						
10. Basketball						
11. Walking						
12. Stair stepper						
13. Swimming						
14. Volleyball						
15. Water polo						
16. Rock climbing	Notes:		Notes:		Notes:	
17. Football						

Daily Fitness Assessment

Total Body Workout

Date _____   Date _____   Date _____

Cardio	#	Time	#	Time	#	Time
1. Stationary Bike						
2. Treadmill						
3. Aerobic classes						
4. Racquetball						
5. Jump rope						
6. Ski machine						
7. Jogging						
8. Jumping jacks						
9. Boxing						
10. Basketball						
11. Walking						
12. Stair stepper						
13. Swimming						
14. Volleyball						
15. Water polo						
16. Rock climbing	Notes:		Notes:		Notes:	
17. Football						

Daily Fitness Assessment

Total Body Workout

	Date _____	Date _____	Date _____

Cardio	#	Time	#	Time	#	Time
1. Stationary Bike						
2. Treadmill						
3. Aerobic classes						
4. Racquetball						
5. Jump rope						
6. Ski machine						
7. Jogging						
8. Jumping jacks						
9. Boxing						
10. Basketball						
11. Walking						
12. Stair stepper						
13. Swimming						
14. Volleyball						
15. Water polo						
16. Rock climbing	Notes:		Notes:		Notes:	
17. Football						

Daily Fitness Assessment

Total Body Workout

Cardio	Date _____		Date _____		Date _____	
	#		#		#	
		Time		Time		Time
1. Stationary Bike						
2. Treadmill						
3. Aerobic classes						
4. Racquetball						
5. Jump rope						
6. Ski machine						
7. Jogging						
8. Jumping jacks						
9. Boxing						
10. Basketball						
11. Walking						
12. Stair stepper						
13. Swimming						
14. Volleyball						
15. Water polo						
16. Rock climbing	Notes:		Notes:		Notes:	
17. Football						

Daily Fitness Assessment

Total Body Workout

	Date _____		Date _____		Date _____	
	#		#		#	
Cardio		Time		Time		Time
1. Stationary Bike						
2. Treadmill						
3. Aerobic classes						
4. Racquetball						
5. Jump rope						
6. Ski machine						
7. Jogging						
8. Jumping jacks						
9. Boxing						
10. Basketball						
11. Walking						
12. Stair stepper						
13. Swimming						
14. Volleyball						
15. Water polo						
16. Rock climbing	Notes:		Notes:		Notes:	
17. Football						

Daily Fitness Assessment

Total Body Workout

	Date _____		Date _____		Date _____	
Cardio	#	Time	#	Time	#	Time
1. Stationary Bike						
2. Treadmill						
3. Aerobic classes						
4. Racquetball						
5. Jump rope						
6. Ski machine						
7. Jogging						
8. Jumping jacks						
9. Boxing						
10. Basketball						
11. Walking						
12. Stair stepper						
13. Swimming						
14. Volleyball						
15. Water polo						
16. Rock climbing	Notes:		Notes:		Notes:	
17. Football						

Daily Fitness Assessment

Total Body Workout

Date _____   Date _____   Date _____

Cardio	#	Time	#	Time	#	Time
1. Stationary Bike						
2. Treadmill						
3. Aerobic classes						
4. Racquetball						
5. Jump rope						
6. Ski machine						
7. Jogging						
8. Jumping jacks						
9. Boxing						
10. Basketball						
11. Walking						
12. Stair stepper						
13. Swimming						
14. Volleyball						
15. Water polo						
16. Rock climbing	Notes:		Notes:		Notes:	
17. Football						

Daily Fitness Assessment

Total Body Workout

	Date _____		Date _____		Date _____	
Cardio	#	Time	#	Time	#	Time
1. Stationary Bike						
2. Treadmill						
3. Aerobic classes						
4. Racquetball						
5. Jump rope						
6. Ski machine						
7. Jogging						
8. Jumping jacks						
9. Boxing						
10. Basketball						
11. Walking						
12. Stair stepper						
13. Swimming						
14. Volleyball						
15. Water polo						
16. Rock climbing	Notes:		Notes:		Notes:	
17. Football						

Daily Fitness Assessment

Total Body Workout

	Date _____		Date _____		Date _____	
Cardio	#	Time	#	Time	#	Time
1. Stationary Bike						
2. Treadmill						
3. Aerobic classes						
4. Racquetball						
5. Jump rope						
6. Ski machine						
7. Jogging						
8. Jumping jacks						
9. Boxing						
10. Basketball						
11. Walking						
12. Stair stepper						
13. Swimming						
14. Volleyball						
15. Water polo						
16. Rock climbing	Notes:		Notes:		Notes:	
17. Football						

Daily Fitness Assessment

Total Body Workout

	Date _____		Date _____		Date _____	
	#		#		#	
Cardio		Time		Time		Time
1. Stationary Bike						
2. Treadmill						
3. Aerobic classes						
4. Racquetball						
5. Jump rope						
6. Ski machine						
7. Jogging						
8. Jumping jacks						
9. Boxing						
10. Basketball						
11. Walking						
12. Stair stepper						
13. Swimming						
14. Volleyball						
15. Water polo						
16. Rock climbing	Notes:		Notes:		Notes:	
17. Football						

Daily Fitness Assessment

Total Body Workout

	Date _____		Date _____		Date _____	
Cardio	#	Time	#	Time	#	Time
1. Stationary Bike						
2. Treadmill						
3. Aerobic classes						
4. Racquetball						
5. Jump rope						
6. Ski machine						
7. Jogging						
8. Jumping jacks						
9. Boxing						
10. Basketball						
11. Walking						
12. Stair stepper						
13. Swimming						
14. Volleyball						
15. Water polo						
16. Rock climbing	Notes:		Notes:		Notes:	
17. Football						

Daily Fitness Assessment

Total Body Workout

Date _____   Date _____   Date _____

Cardio	#	Time	#	Time	#	Time
1. Stationary Bike						
2. Treadmill						
3. Aerobic classes						
4. Racquetball						
5. Jump rope						
6. Ski machine						
7. Jogging						
8. Jumping jacks						
9. Boxing						
10. Basketball						
11. Walking						
12. Stair stepper						
13. Swimming						
14. Volleyball						
15. Water polo						
16. Rock climbing	Notes:		Notes:		Notes:	
17. Football